HERBAL ADAPTOGENS FOR LONGITIVITY

Harnessing Nature's Power, A Guide To Lasting Healthier Life

DR. JEREMY ALLEY

1

Copyright © JEREMY ALLEY 2024

Disclaimer:

The information provided in this book, is intended for general informational purposes only and should not be considered as professional advice.

The author has made every effort to ensure the accuracy of the information presented. However, readers are advised to consult with a qualified healthcare professional before attempting any herbal remedies or making significant changes to their wellness routine. Individual health conditions vary, and what may be suitable for one person may not be appropriate for another.

It is important to note that the author is not in any endorsement deal, partnership, or affiliation with any organization, brand, or company mentioned in this book. Any references to specific products or services are based on the author's personal experience or general knowledge and do not imply an endorsement or promotion of those products or services.

Contents

Introduction

People typically look into different ways to improve their health and live longer in an attempt to live longer. Of all the several strategies, using herbal adaptogens has drawn the most attention because of its potential benefits for extending life. The purpose of this book is to examine the world of herbal adaptogens, including their characteristics, workings, and role in promoting lifespan. Through comprehending the mutually beneficial connection between adaptogenic herbs and the human body, readers can acquire knowledge about integrating these organic treatments into their daily routines.

About The Book

A family of botanicals known for their capacity to support the body's ability to maintain equilibrium and adjust to stimuli is known as herbal adaptogens. These herbs, which have their roots in traditional medical systems like Ayurveda and Traditional Chinese Medicine, have been used for centuries to promote resilience and general health. An overview of popular adaptogens will be given in this part, along with information on their historical use, scientific underpinnings, and places of origin. Readers will acquire a basic understanding of the wide variety of herbs that fall under the umbrella term "adaptogen."

The Idea of Lifespan

The goal of living a longer and healthier life is known as longevity, and it has always been ingrained in human civilization. This section will examine lifespan from scientific, cultural, and historical angles. By exploring the variables that affect lifespan, such as genetic predispositions and lifestyle decisions, readers will have a thorough grasp of what makes for a longer, more satisfying life. The conversation will also touch on how society is changing its views on aging and how herbal adaptogens can help in the pursuit of longer life spans.

Goals and Purpose of the Book

This book is meant to be a thorough reference for anyone interested in using herbal adaptogens to improve their health and lengthen their life.

The processes by which adaptogens interact with the body's stress response systems will be clarified, giving readers the information they need to make wise decisions regarding their health.

 The scope looks at the special qualities and possible advantages of a wide variety of adaptogenic plants.

Furthermore, useful advice and suggestions for incorporating adaptogens into everyday living will be given, giving readers concrete ways to start along the path to a longer and better life.

CHAPTER ONE

RECOGNIZING ADAPTOGENS

In the field of holistic health, adaptogens—a family of herbs known for their capacity to strengthen the body's resistance to stress—have drawn a lot of interest.

These remarkable botanicals are distinguished by their special qualities that support general well-being by assisting the body in adapting to a variety of stimuli.

This section explores the meaning and properties of adaptogens, providing insight into their historical application and the complex mechanisms underlying their amazing benefits.

Definition And Qualities

By definition, adaptogens are organic compounds that help the body maintain physiological balance while adjusting to stimuli. These amazing herbs are non-specific, which means they can influence how the body reacts to stimuli without interfering with regular biological processes.

What makes adaptogens unique is their capacity to offer a broad defense against a variety of stressors—chemical, biological, or physical—without endangering health or generating imbalance.

One of the adaptogens' qualities is their nonspecificity, which allows them to promote the body's resilience without focusing on a particular organ or system.

Moreover, these herbs have a normalizing effect that aids in reestablishing the equilibrium of the body's physiological processes.

Furthermore, well-known for their low toxicity, adaptogens are usually safe to use over an extended period.

Adaptogens have been used historically in traditional medical systems across many cultures. Adaptogenic herbs have long been used in traditional medicine practices by indigenous cultures worldwide.

Adaptogens such as holy basil and ashwagandha are prized in Ayurveda, the traditional Indian medical system, for their capacity to increase energy and lengthen life.

Similar to this, adaptogenic herbs like ginseng and rhodiola have long been used in Traditional Chinese Medicine (TCM) to boost the body's ability to withstand stress.

For many years, indigenous cultures in Scandinavia, Russia, and other areas have also used the adaptogens found in the native flora.

The various ways that adaptogens work to benefit the body are closely related to the systems that regulate the body's stress response.

The control of the hypothalamic-pituitary-adrenal (HPA) axis, a vital part of the body's stress response, is one of the main mechanisms. Adaptogens support a more balanced and adaptive response to stimuli by regulating the production of stress hormones like cortisol.

Furthermore, adaptogens increase the body's cellular energy generation and facilitate the effective use of resources during stressful times. Additionally, these herbs have antioxidant properties that shield cells from stress-related oxidative damage.

The immune system's and neurotransmitters' regulation adds to the adaptogens' all-encompassing advantages by impacting both physical and mental health.

Gaining knowledge about these complex pathways of action can help us better understand how adaptogens affect longevity and general health.

In the search for herbal remedies that enhance resilience and longevity, adaptogens are an interesting field of study due to the combination of these properties.

CHAPTER TWO

THE LONGEVITY SCIENCE

The desire to live a longer and healthier life has always been a universal human goal. When we dig deeper into the details of this intricate idea, we find that several things affect people's general health and longer life expectancy.

The study of longevity covers a wide range of factors that affect how long we live, from genetic predispositions to lifestyle decisions.

Factors Influencing Lifespan

Examining the various elements that influence aging is necessary to comprehend the complex relationship between longevity and various circumstances.

Factors including as genetics, dietary habits, exercise habits, stress levels, and environmental exposures are significant determinants of how gracefully people age. Every component affects the general health and lifespan of an individual by interacting with others in a dynamic and interwoven web.

Deciphering the complexities of these elements offers important information for developing tactics that encourage living longer and in better health.

Adaptogens' Function In Anti-Aging

Adaptogens are interesting ingredients that may help promote anti-aging benefits in the quest for longevity. Herbal medical systems have long employed a class of plants known as adaptogens, most notably Ayurveda and Traditional Chinese medicine.

These herbs have special qualities that support the body's ability to adjust to both internal and external stimuli. Adaptogens' capacity to regulate the stress response is becoming more widely acknowledged as a critical component in the search for anti-aging remedies.

Adaptogens influence the body's primary stress response mechanism, the hypothalamic-pituitary-adrenal (HPA) axis, which helps control the release of stress hormones like cortisol.

Adaptogens support resilience and equilibrium in the face of stress, which enhances people's general well-being. It is believed that this adaptogenic balance goes beyond only relieving stress right away; it may also slow down aging and lengthen life.

Research On The Longevity Of Herbs In Science

An increasing amount of scientific evidence supports the use of adaptogens in the quest for longevity.

Several research works have investigated the bioactive substances found in different adaptogenic herbs and their possible influence on processes associated with aging.

Scholars have examined the anti-inflammatory, immunomodulatory, and antioxidant characteristics of these herbs to decipher the molecular processes that underlie their benefits on longevity.

Studies on the longevity of herbs frequently concentrate on certain adaptogens, such as holy basil, ashwagandha, Panax ginseng, Rhodiola rosea, and others.

These studies explore the herb's capacity to assist cellular repair pathways, lessen inflammation, and decrease oxidative stress.

The results of these investigations provide important new information on the possible function of adaptogens in enhancing longevity and good aging.

A comprehensive grasp of the variables impacting the aging process is included in the science of longevity.

Studies have shown that adaptogens play a fascinating role in anti-aging and provide insight into the methods by which these herbal treatments might prolong and improve one's life expectancy. The possibility of combining these herbs into holistic treatments for aging looks more and more intriguing as the research unfolds the complex relationships between adaptogens and longevity.

CHAPTER THREE

PREVIOUS ADAPTOGENS HERBS

Rose Rhodiola

Golden root, or Rhodiola Rosea, is a highly esteemed adaptogen with a long history of application in conventional medicine.

This herb, which is native to the arctic regions of Europe and Asia, has been linked to higher resilience to stress, increased stamina, and improved mental clarity.

Due to its adaptogenic qualities, it is a well-liked option for people looking to live long and vibrant lives.

Ashwagandha

A common ingredient in Ayurvedic medicine, ashwagandha is well known for its restorative qualities. Ashwagandha, sometimes called "Indian ginseng," has been used traditionally to support energy, reduce stress, and improve general vitality. Its adaptogenic properties encourage a healthy stress response and may prolong and improve overall health.

Sacred Basil (Tulsi)

In Ayurveda, holy basil, or tulsi, is revered as a sacred herb. Respected for its healing and adaptogenic properties, tulsi is said to lengthen life by lowering inflammation and stress levels in the body. Holy basil has earned a spot among the best adaptogens for people looking for a holistic approach to well-being because of its balancing and relaxing properties.

Ginseng

In traditional Chinese and Native American medicine, ginseng—more specifically, Panax ginseng and Panax quinquefolius, or Asian and

American ginseng, respectively—is a well-known adaptogen. Ginseng is well known for boosting immunity, increasing vitality, and enhancing cognitive function.

Its reputation as a herb that might promote a longer, better life is mostly due to these characteristics.

Eleuthero Ginseng From Siberia

Siberian ginseng, or eleuthero, has long been a part of traditional Chinese and Russian medicine. This adaptogen has been linked to greater general resilience to stress, improved immunological function, and higher endurance.

Eleuthero is still a well-liked option for people looking for natural ways to enhance their well-being because it may contribute to longevity.

Berry Schisandra

Native to China and Russia, the schisandra berry is a special adaptogen with five distinct flavors: sweet, sour, salty, bitter, and pungent. It is thought to lengthen life and tonify the body's life force in traditional Chinese medicine. Schisandra's adaptogenic qualities are believed to support the body's ability to adjust to stimuli and maintain a resilient, balanced condition.

Maral Root, Rhaponticum Carthamoides

Native to Siberia, Rhaponticum carthamoides is often referred to as Maral Root. It is an adaptogenic herb. Maral Root has been used traditionally to improve mental and physical performance. It is said to prolong longevity by enhancing the body's ability to adapt to stress. Potential advantages include heightened vitality, elevated mood, and enhanced general well-being.

Including herbal adaptogens in one's diet could provide a holistic, all-natural means of extending life. Many traditional and contemporary applications can be found for the adaptogenic herbs Rhodiola Rosea, Ashwagandha, Holy Basil, Ginseng, Eleuthero, Schisandra Berry, and Rhaponticum Carthamoides.

Although individual results may differ, conventional medicine's body of knowledge indicates that these adaptogens are important for bolstering the body's resilience and may even help people live longer, healthier lives.

CHAPTER FOUR

COMPOSING ADAPTIVE BLENDS

Adaptogens have drawn a lot of interest because of their possible ability to extend life and improve general well-being.

These herbs are essential for supporting many physiological processes and are well-known for their capacity to assist the body in adapting to stressors. Creating adaptogenic blends entails blending particular herbs to maximize their advantages and strengthen their synergistic effects.

Combinations That Work Together

Blending adaptogens necessitates a thorough comprehension of the unique characteristics and possible interactions of each herb.

Certain herbs have synergistic effects that amplify their adaptogenic qualities when combined. For instance, mixing Panax ginseng with Rhodiola rosea may provide a more thorough stress-adaptation response. Herbalists and formulators can produce blends that target specific health concerns and individual needs by experimenting with different combinations and ratios.

Administration & Dosage

One of the most important aspects of adaptogenic blends' effectiveness is figuring out how to administer and dose them correctly. The ideal dosage can change depending on a person's weight, age, and general health.

To see how the body reacts, it is crucial to begin with lesser doses and raise them gradually. Certain adaptogens might work better in the morning, while others would work better in the evening. Developing an efficient dosage plan requires knowledge of each herb's unique adaptogenic qualities as well as the circadian rhythm.

Possible Reactions With Medications And Other Herbs

Although adaptogens are usually thought to be safe, it's important to be aware of any potential interactions, particularly when taking them with other drugs or plants.

Before adding adaptogenic blends to their regimen, people should speak with healthcare providers, especially if they are already taking medication, as some adaptogens may increase or decrease the effects of certain medications.

To guarantee the safe incorporation of adaptogens into a comprehensive health routine, it is imperative to keep an eye out for any unanticipated consequences or negative reactions.

When carefully chosen and used, adaptogens can be effective allies in fostering longevity and fortitude in the face of adversity.

Creating adaptogenic blends requires a careful balancing act between knowing the unique properties of each plant, investigating synergistic combinations, figuring out the best dosages, and being aware of any possible conflicts with other drugs and herbs.

People can use adaptogens to support their overall health and lifespan by combining these herbs into a complete wellness program.

CHAPTER FIVE

FORMULATING LONGEVITY ELIXIRS

The use of adaptogens in daily routines has garnered considerable interest in the quest for a life that is both healthier and more resilient.

These herbal medicines are essential for increasing longevity because of their capacity to support general well-being, assist the body in adjusting to stress, and both.

This investigation explores a variety of longevity elixir recipes, providing a wide array of delectable and health-promoting concoctions that integrate adaptogens.

Blends Of Adaptogenic Teas

Tea is a great beverage to add adaptogens to because of its variety of flavors and cozy warmth. The technique of creating adaptogenic tea blends— which enhance the body's resistance while simultaneously calming the senses—is examined in this section.

These adaptogenic tea blends, which range from traditional concoctions like holy basil and ashwagandha to creative infusions like rhodiola and licorice root, are designed to promote longevity by establishing a harmonious equilibrium.

Recipes For Smoothies And Juices

Smoothies and juices are a tasty method to absorb adaptogens for people who prefer a liquid approach to wellness.

This section includes several recipes that use adaptogenic herbs to create delectable drinks. Whether it's a revitalizing juice combination with Schisandra and Astragalus or a cool green smoothie with maca and spirulina, these recipes offer a delicious and practical way to take advantage of adaptogens' ability to extend life.

Infusions And Tinctures

Strong herbal medicines such as tinctures and infusions provide concentrated dosages of adaptogens. The technique of making tinctures and infusions that are simple to adopt into every day routines is covered in this section. These preparations, which range from a ginseng and eleuthero infusion that boosts vitality to a relaxing lavender and reishi tincture, provide a focused and practical approach to incorporating adaptogens into one's wellness program.

Including Adaptogens In Regular Foods

When adaptogens are incorporated into regular meals, commonplace foods become effective instruments for extending life. This section offers tips for preparing a wide range of dishes, from savory soups to sweet confections, using adaptogens. Find out how to improve the nutritional profile of your meals by preparing your favorite foods with adaptogenic spices like ashwagandha or adding adaptogenic mushrooms like chaga.

The goal of these culinary inventions is to include the benefits of adaptogens—which promote longevity—into your regular diet.

Ultimately, we want to enjoy the union of flavor and health as we proceed through these recipes for longevity elixirs.

Every segment presents a distinct viewpoint on integrating adaptogens into various aspects of our everyday existence, promoting a comprehensive strategy for well-being and longevity.

CHAPTER SIX

LIFESTYLE ACTIONS TO ENHANCE LIVING

Taking up different activities that enhance general health is part of living a long-lived lifestyle. One important component is stress management, which is essential for increasing longevity and the body's resistance to adversity.

Techniques For Stress Management

Prolonged stress can have detrimental effects on one's physical and emotional well-being, possibly shortening one's lifespan.

Using stress-reduction strategies is crucial to reducing these impacts. The body's stress reaction can be controlled with the aid of techniques like progressive muscle relaxation, biofeedback, and deep breathing exercises.

Strong social ties and keeping a support network can also serve as a stress-reduction strategy. Engaging in joyful hobbies, socializing, and spending time with loved ones all support emotional well-being, which is strongly associated with longevity.

Optimizing Sleep

A long and healthy life is mostly dependent on getting enough good quality sleep, which is also linked to lifespan.

A class of herbs called adaptogens, which are well-known for reducing stress, may help to improve sleep. Herbs known to be adaptogenic, such as holy basil and ashwagandha, have long been used to help the body adjust to stressors and enhance the quality of sleep.

Essential elements of sleep optimization include establishing a sleep-friendly atmosphere, keeping to a regular sleep schedule, and engaging in relaxation exercises before to going to bed. These routines enhance general longevity and promote a good night's sleep, especially when paired with some herbs' adaptogenic qualities.

Exercise Physically

Frequent exercise is a reliable indicator of longevity. Exercise improves mood and cognitive performance in addition to helping one maintain a healthy weight and cardiovascular system. Including adaptogens in one's regimen can enhance the advantages of physical activity by mitigating the oxidative stress linked to it.

Herbs known to be adaptogenic, such as ginseng and rhodiola, have been researched for their ability to improve physical performance overall, lessen fatigue, and increase endurance. Including these herbs in a comprehensive exercise program can enhance the benefits of regular exercise on longevity.

Meditation And Mindfulness

The benefits of mindfulness techniques, such as meditation, on mental health and general wellbeing have come to light.

These effects can be increased by using adaptogenic herbs in mindfulness practices. Herbs that are traditionally used to strengthen cognitive function and improve mental clarity include eleuthero and tulsi, sometimes known as holy basil.

Using adaptogens with mindfulness meditation can be especially beneficial for lowering stress and fostering emotional resilience.

This synergistic approach emphasizes the connection between the mind and body by addressing both the psychological and physiological components of lifespan.

Longevity can be achieved by implementing a lifestyle that emphasizes stress reduction, sleep hygiene, consistent exercise, and mindfulness exercises.

These lifestyle habits can be made even more effective by including adaptogenic herbs, which offer a comprehensive strategy for fostering general well-being and a longer, healthier life.

CHAPTER SEVEN

MENTAL WELL-BEING AND HERBAL ADAPTOGENS

The potential of herbal adaptogens to support longevity and mental well-being has drawn a lot of interest.

These organic compounds, which come from a variety of plants, have special qualities that support the body's ability to adjust to both physical and psychological stimuli.

This article examines how herbal adaptogens affect mental health, with particular attention to mental clarity, anxiety, depression, and cognitive performance.

Brain Activity And Adaptogens

Boosting cognitive function is one of the main areas where herbal adaptogens show their effectiveness. Studies have looked into the potential of adaptogenic herbs, like Rhodiola rosea and Panax ginseng, to improve memory, focus, and general cognitive function. These herbs are thought to support optimum brain function and regulate the release of stress hormones, which enhances cognitive ability.

Handling Depression And Anxiety

Moreover, adaptogens have demonstrated promise in treating anxiety and depressive symptoms. Long-term stress can negatively impact mental health and contribute to disorders like depression and anxiety.

Traditionally, herbs like holy basil (tulsi) and ashwagandha have been utilized to reduce anxiety and tension.

According to scientific research, these adaptogens may affect brain neurotransmitters including serotonin and gamma-aminobutyric acid (GABA), which may help maintain a more stable mood.

Improving Emotional Intelligence

Herbal adaptogens are known to support mental clarity in addition to alleviating mood disorders and promoting cognitive function.

The potential of adaptogens to regulate stress responses could be a factor in decreased cognitive fog and enhanced concentration.

Herbs with neuroprotective qualities, such as Bacopa monnieri, are thought to support brain health in general and cognitive clarity in particular, making them valuable additions to formulations meant to promote mental acuity.

Herbal Blends For All-Around Mental Support

Blending different adaptogenic herbs can have a synergistic impact for all-encompassing mental support. Herbal formulations that incorporate a variety of adaptogens with complementary qualities may give a holistic approach to mental well-being.

A combination of herbs, such as Bacopa monnieri for mental clarity, Ashwagandha for stress relief, and Rhodiola rosea for cognitive enhancement, may be able to address several aspects of mental health and encourage resilience in the face of a variety of stressors.

Individual Variability And Herbal Adaptogens

It's vital to note that individual responses to herbal adaptogens can differ. Factors such as genetics, lifestyle, and overall health play a role in determining how a person responds to these natural remedies.

While some individuals may experience significant benefits, others might have a more subtle response. Consulting with a healthcare professional before incorporating adaptogens into one's routine is advisable, especially for those with pre-existing medical conditions or those taking medication.

herbal adaptogens offer a promising avenue for promoting mental well-being and longevity. Their impact on cognitive function, anxiety, depression, and mental clarity highlights their diverse benefits. As interest in natural approaches to mental health continues to grow, further research into the mechanisms and optimal combinations of adaptogenic herbs may provide valuable insights for both preventive and therapeutic applications.

As with any supplement or herbal remedy, individual considerations and professional guidance should be taken into account for a personalized and safe approach to mental wellness.

CHAPTER EIGHT

LONGEVITY IN TRADITIONAL MEDICINE SYSTEMS

Longevity has been a pursuit of humanity throughout history, and traditional medicine systems have played a significant role in this quest. Various cultures around the world have developed unique approaches to promoting longevity, often incorporating herbal adaptogens into their practices. This article explores the use of herbal adaptogens in traditional medicine systems, focusing on Ayurveda, Traditional Chinese Medicine (TCM), and indigenous medicinal practices.

Ayurveda And Adaptogens

Ayurveda, the ancient system of medicine originating from India, places a strong emphasis on achieving balance in the body and mind.

Ayurvedic practitioners have long recognized the potential of adaptogenic herbs in promoting longevity.

Adaptogens, such as Ashwagandha and Holy Basil (Tulsi), are integral components of Ayurvedic formulations aimed at enhancing vitality and resilience.

These herbs are believed to strengthen the body's response to stress, support immune function, and contribute to overall well-being, ultimately fostering a longer and healthier life.

Traditional Chinese Medicine And Longevity Herbs

Traditional Chinese Medicine has a rich history that spans thousands of years, and the pursuit of longevity has been a central theme in this ancient system. Chinese herbal medicine incorporates a variety of adaptogens known for their potential to promote longevity.

Herbs like Panax ginseng, Astragalus, and Rhodiola are frequently used in TCM formulations aimed at supporting vital energy, nourishing the body, and promoting a balanced and harmonious life force. These adaptogens are believed to strengthen the body's resilience and contribute to a longer and healthier life according to the principles of TCM.

Indigenous Medicinal Practices

Indigenous cultures around the world have developed unique medicinal practices based on local flora and traditional knowledge. These practices often include the use of adaptogenic herbs that are believed to contribute to longevity.

From the Amazon rainforest to the Arctic tundra, indigenous communities have identified plants with adaptogenic properties, incorporating them into their healing traditions.

The knowledge of these herbs is passed down through generations, forming an integral part of the cultural and spiritual fabric of these communities.

The use of adaptogens in indigenous medicinal practices reflects a holistic approach to health and longevity, addressing the interconnectedness of the individual with their environment.

As we delve into the intricate web of traditional medicine systems and their use of herbal adaptogens for longevity, it becomes evident that these practices are deeply rooted in a holistic understanding of the human body, mind, and spirit. The diverse array of adaptogenic herbs employed in Ayurveda, Traditional Chinese Medicine, and indigenous medicinal practices underscores the universal human quest for a longer and healthier life.

Through the ages, these traditional systems have provided insights into the potential of nature's remedies to support well-being and promote longevity, offering valuable lessons that continue to resonate in our modern world.

CHAPTER NINE

SUCCESS STORIES AND CASE STUDIES

Real-life experiences serve as compelling evidence of the efficacy of herbal adaptogens in promoting longevity. This section features case studies and success stories, showcasing individuals who have incorporated adaptogens into their lives and witnessed positive impacts on their overall well-being.

Testimonials And Anecdotes

Testimonials and anecdotes from individuals who have embraced herbal adaptogens provide a personal dimension to the exploration of longevity benefits. By sharing their experiences, these individuals offer valuable insights into the diverse ways adaptogens may contribute to enhanced resilience and a longer, healthier life.

Risks And Considerations

Before incorporating herbal adaptogens into a wellness regimen, it's crucial to be aware of potential risks and considerations. This section provides a comprehensive overview, covering areas such as potential side effects, contraindications, and safety guidelines. Understanding these aspects is essential for making informed decisions about the use of herbal adaptogens for longevity.

Potential Side Effects

While herbal adaptogens are generally considered safe, there may be potential side effects associated with their use. This section explores the reported side effects of popular adaptogens and discusses factors that may influence individual responses. It emphasizes the importance of monitoring for adverse reactions and consulting with a healthcare professional if necessary.

Contraindications

Certain populations and individuals with specific health conditions may need to exercise caution or avoid certain herbal adaptogens. This section outlines contraindications, offering guidance on who should approach these herbs with care. It emphasizes the importance of consulting with a healthcare provider, especially for those with pre-existing medical conditions or taking medications.

Safety Guidelines

To ensure the safe and effective use of herbal adaptogens, adherence to safety guidelines is paramount.

This section provides practical advice on selecting high-quality products, determining appropriate dosages, and monitoring for any adverse reactions.

Emphasizing the importance of a balanced approach, these guidelines aim to support individuals in incorporating herbal adaptogens into their lifestyles responsibly.

CONCLUSION

the exploration of herbal adaptogens for longevity reveals a fascinating intersection of traditional wisdom and modern scientific inquiry.

The adaptogenic properties of these herbs, combined with a growing body of research, suggest that they may play a valuable role in supporting a long and healthy life.

As individuals seek holistic approaches to well-being, incorporating herbal adaptogens into their lifestyle holds promise for promoting resilience and longevity.

Summary Of Important Ideas

A brief recapitulation of the key points reinforces the core concepts discussed in this article. From the definition of adaptogens to their mechanisms of action and the exploration of specific herbs, this recap serves as a quick reference for readers seeking to consolidate their understanding of the role of herbal adaptogens in longevity.

Looking Forward To A Long And Healthy Life

The final section looks ahead to the potential future developments in the field of herbal adaptogens and longevity. As research continues and more people recognize the importance of holistic health practices, the integration of adaptogens into mainstream wellness routines may become more widespread. Embracing a proactive approach to health, individuals can look forward to a future characterized by vitality, resilience, and an enhanced quality of life.